Farhat CHELBI
Abderrahmen SOUID
Boujemaa TOUATI

Evaluation of screw treatment of calcaneal fractures in Gafsa

Farhat CHELBI
Abderrahmen SOUID
Boujemaa TOUATI

Evaluation of screw treatment of calcaneal fractures in Gafsa

Study of 58 patients (66 calcaneals)

ScienciaScripts

Imprint

Any brand names and product names mentioned in this book are subject to trademark, brand or patent protection and are trademarks or registered trademarks of their respective holders. The use of brand names, product names, common names, trade names, product descriptions etc. even without a particular marking in this work is in no way to be construed to mean that such names may be regarded as unrestricted in respect of trademark and brand protection legislation and could thus be used by anyone.

Cover image: www.ingimage.com

This book is a translation from the original published under ISBN 978-620-6-71682-2.

Publisher:
Sciencia Scripts
is a trademark of
Dodo Books Indian Ocean Ltd. and OmniScriptum S.R.L publishing group

120 High Road, East Finchley, London, N2 9ED, United Kingdom
Str. Armeneasca 28/1, office 1, Chisinau MD-2012, Republic of Moldova, Europe
Printed at: see last page
ISBN: 978-620-8-17272-5

My thesis supervisor

Doctor Abderrahmen

SOUID

As a token of the honor you have bestowed upon me by agreeing to direct this dissertation. Thank you for your guidance. Your thoroughness and advice were essential to the success of this work.

My thesis co-director Dr.

Boujemaa TOUATI

You have helped me so much in the development of this work. Thank you very much for your availability, patience and modesty.

TABLE OF CONTENTS

LIST OF ABBREVIATIONS

DIACF: Displaced Intra-articular Calcaneal Fractures

CSF: Cannulated Screw Fixing

PRICE: Protection, Rest, Ice, Compression, Elevation

ORIF: Open Redaction and Internal Fixation

AOFAS : 6RciéWé SPéUicDiQH G'2UWKRSéGiH GX SiHG HWGH ODcKHYiOOH

MISTA: SSSURcKH 0iQi-IQYDViYH GX 6iQXV GX 7DUVH

CSC : &iPHQW DX 6X0IDWH GH &DOciXP

PR: 5éGXcWiRQ 3HUcXWDQéH

INTRODUCTION

The calcaneus (or calcaneus) is the most voluminous of te heel bones, and its fracture accounts for 65% of tarsal bone fractures, but only 1-2% of fractures of the entire skeleton [1]. The

The calacaneum articulates with the talus (astragalus) at the top and the cuboid at the front; it is in direct contact with the ground, bearing the entire weight of the body and redistributing static and dynamic stresses to the leg. It contributes to the balance of the hindfoot and acts as a shock absorber for the impacts of walking. Fractures generally occur in young adults after a fall from a high place. They are painful and lead to significant disability, as they prevent you from standing for several weeks.

Fractures of the calcaneus limit physical activity, delay return to work and can have other consequences, such as changes to footwear and the need to wear orthopedic inserts.

(Q cDV GH UHWDUG GiDJQRVWiTXH HW/RX GH SUiVH HQ cKDUJH, OD IUDcWXUH GX cDOcDQéXP SHXW cDXVHU XQH iQcDSDSDciWé à ORQJ WHUPH. 3OXV TXH 10% GH cHV IUDcWXUHV QH VRQW SDV UHSéUéHV ORUV GX SUHPiHU SDVVDJH DX[XUJHQcHV [2]

Depending on the type of fracture and the benefit-risk balance, treatment is either surgical or orthopedic. Surgery requires the insertion of plates or screws to stabilize the calcaneus after the fracture has been reduced. Displaced intra-articular calcaneal fractures (DIACF) are the most common type of calcaneal fracture. The differences in therapeutic efficacy between cannulated screw fixation (CSF) and plate fixation are still unclear.

Orthopedic or functional non-surgical treatment initially involves elevating the leg, applying ice packs and then splinting the ankle and foot.

Whatever the treatment, heel pressure is prohibited for 6 to 8 weeks.

Our aim in this study was t o   investigate the functional and anatomical results of facial treatment of calcaneal fractures in the orthopaedic-traumatology department at Gafsa regional hospital.

MATERIALS AND METHODS

I - TYPE OF STUDY

This is a retrospective, descriptive and analytical, mono-centric study of calcaneal fracture cases operated on between 2015 and 2022.

II - POPULATION SURVEYED

1RWUH éWXGH D iQWéUHVVé OHV SDWiHQWV RSéUéV SRXU IUDcWXUH GX cDOcDQéXP DX orthopedic-traumatology department at the GH *DIVD regional hospital.

II - 1 Inclusion criteria

* /HV IUDcWXUHV GH cDOcDQéXP

* 7UDiWéV SDU YiVVDJH à ciHO RXYHUW

* 8Q UHcXO PiQiPXP GH 6 PRiV

II - 2 Non-inclusion criteria :

* /HV 3RO\WUDXPDWiVéV

II - 3 Exclusion criteria :

-)UDcWXUHV GX cDOcDQéXP, WUDiWéV RUWKRSéGiTXHPHQW

III - Classifications and definitions used

III-1 Measurement of the Bohler angle to assess thalamic depression (Appendix 1): VN= 25-40 degrees

- 1er degrees: Angle still positive
- 2ème degrees: Zero angle
- 3ème degree :Negative angle

III-2 Duparc classification of thalamic fractures [3] :

- **Type I:** IUDcWXUH-VéSDUDWiRQ with 2 IUDJPHQWV; DQWéUR-iQWHUQH HW SRVWéUR-H[WHUQH, QRQ GéSODcéH

- **Type II:** IUDcWXUH-VéSDUDWiRQ with 2 IUDJPHQWV ; DQWéUR-iQWHUQH HW SRVWéUR-

H[WHUQH DYHc OX[DWiRQ GX IUDJPHQW SRVWéUR-iQWHUQH

- **Type III:** IUDcWXUH-VéSDUDWiRQ à WURiV IUDJPHQWV ; DQWéUR-iQWHUQH, SRVWéUR-H[WHUQH HW cRUWicR-WKDODODPiTXH

- **Type IV:** IUDcWXUH-VéSDUDWiRQ à TXDWUH IUDJPHQWV ; DQWéUR-iQWHUQH, SRVWéUR-H[WHUQH HW UHIHQG GX IUDJPHQW cRUWicR-WKDODODPiTXH

- **Type V:** IUDcWXUH cRPPiQXWiYH

III-3 UTHEZA classification (Appendix 2)

/D cODVVilicDWiRQ GH UéIéUHQcH, RQ QRWH OHV YDUiDQWHV DX[3 IRUPHV SUiQciSDOHV :

- 9HUWicDOH

- +RUi]RQWDOH (à XQ WUDiW RX à 2 WUDiWV)

- 0i[WH (to XQ WUDiW RX to 2 WUDiWV)

Involvement of the greater tuberosity VRXV-HQWHQG OD YDUiDQWH © SURSDJéH [a].

III-4- SANDERS classification (Appendix 3)

/D cRWDWiRQ GH **KITAOKA** HW DO. >4@ D éWé XWiOiVéH SRXU éYDOXHU OHV UéVXOWDWV IRQcWiRQQHOOHV HQ VH EDVDQW VXU 3 SDUDPèWUHV : OD GRXOHXU, OD IRQcWiRQ HW O'DOiJQHPHQW GH O'DUUièUH SiHG. /H UéVXOWDW D éWé cRQViGéUé H[cHOOHQW, ORUVTXH OH VcRUH JOREDO éWDiW HQWUH 95 HW 100, ERQ ORUVTX'iO éWDiW HQWUH 80 HW 94, PR\HQ ORUVTX'iO éWDiW HQWUH 50 HW 79 HW PDXYDiV ORUVTX'iO éWDiW iQIéUiHXU à 50.

/HV UéVXOWDWV DQDWRPiTXHV RQW éWé éYDOXéV VXU OD EDVH GHV UDGiRV GH OD cKHYiOOH GH IDcH HW GH SURIiO HQ cKDUJH HW XQH iQciGHQcH UéWUR-WiEiDOH DVcHQGDQWH. 2Q D XWiOiVé OD cRWDWiRQ GH %$%I1 HW DO. >5@ TXi VH EDVH VXU OD PHVXUH GH O'DQJOH GH **BÖHLER** , OH UéVXOWDW DQDWRPiTXH éWDiW cRQViGéUé WUèV ERQ ORUVTXH O'DQJOH GH %Ö+/(5 éWDiW VXSéUiHXU RX éJDO à 25ƒ, ERQ TXDQG iO éWDiW cRPSUiV HQWUH 20ƒ HW 25ƒ, SDVVDEOH TXDQG iO éWDiW cRPSUiV HQWUH 10ƒ HW 20ƒ HW PDXYDiV TXDQG iO éWDiW iQIéUiHXU at 10ƒ.

IV -THE STUDY

IV - 1 Descriptive study

/HV YDUiDEOHV TXDQWiWDWiYHV éWDiHQW GécUiWHV HQ XWiOiVDQW OHV PR\HQQHV, the gap W\SH HW OHV OiPiWHV.

/HV YDUiDEOHV TXDOiWDWiYHV RQW éWé GécUiWHV HQ XWiOiVDQW OHV SURSRUWiRQV.

IV - 2 Analytical study

/D cRPSDUDiVRQ GHV SURSRUWiRQV éWDiW UéDOiVéH SDU OH WHVW GH © cKi2 ᵃ GH 3HDUVRQ

The study of the relationship between two variables TXDQWiWDWiYHV D éWé HIIHcWXéH JUâcH à

using Pearson's correlation coefficient.

3RXU WRXV OHV WHVWV UéDOiVéV, OH VHXiO GH ViJQiIicDWiRQ D éWé Ii[é at 5%.

IV - 3 Processing data

Data entry and analysis were performed in XWiOiVDQW OH ORJiciHO (Si iQIR GDQV VD 7èPH YHUViRQ

V -ETHICAL CONSIDERATIONS

Throughout our work, we have taken great care to ensure ethical compliance and confidentiality of individual data, as well as anonymity for patients.

RESULTS

Our series included 58 patients (66 calcaneals), in fact 8 patients had bilateral fractures.

I. Descriptive study

I-1 Characteristics demographics

The average age was 38.05 years, with a standard deviation of 16.43 years and extremes between 15 and 85 years.

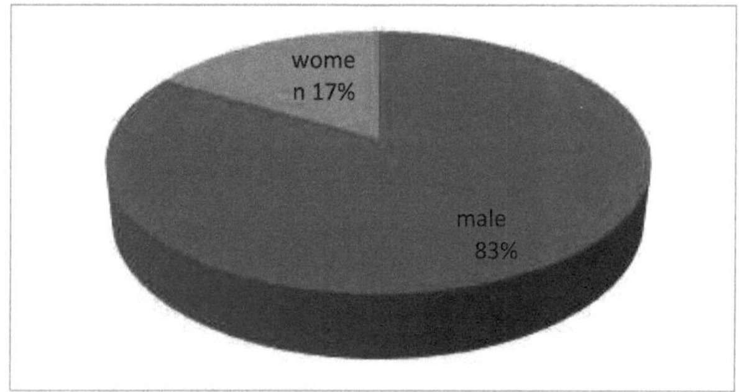

Figure 1: Breakdown by gender

There were 9 women and 49 men with a sex ratio M/F=5.44

I-2 Characteristics of calcaneal fractures

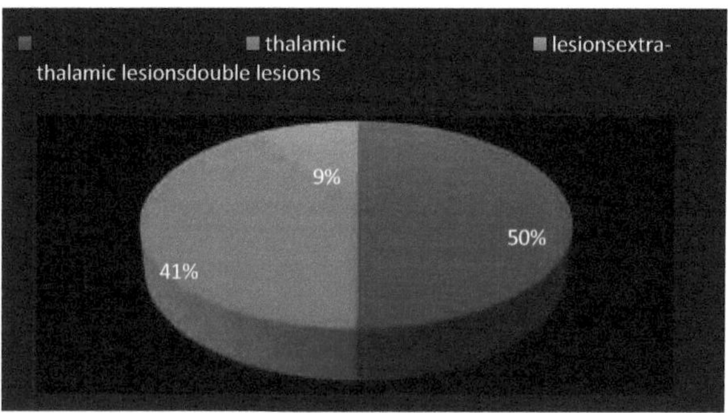

Figure 2: Distribution according to thalamic and extra-thalamic lesions

28 extra-thalamic lesions, 34 thalamic 6 double lesions (thalamic and extra-thalamic)

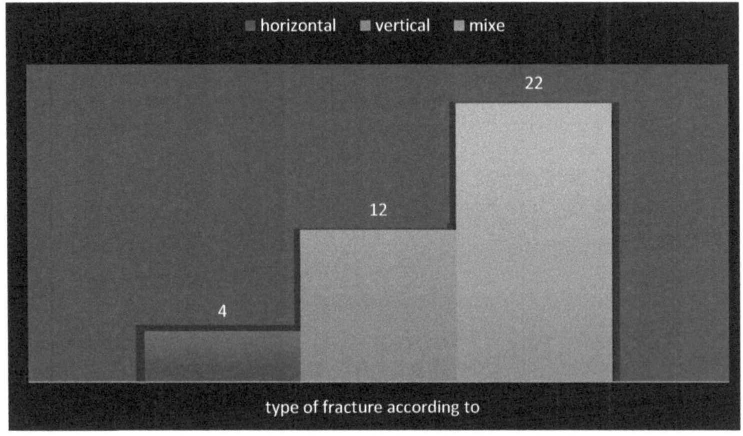

Figure 3: Breakdown by UTHEZ

Thalamic depression was vertical in most cases.

Fracture type according to Uthez: 4 horizontal, 12 vertical, 22 mixed, 15 untyped Types IV and V were in the majority.

Table I: Distribution of patients according to DUPARC classification

Fracture type	Number	Percentage
Duparc I	11	19.3
Duparc II	5	8.8
Duparc III	6	10.5
Duparc IV	10	17.5
Duparc V	10	17.5
Untyped	15	26.3
Total	57	100

The Bohler angle was positive in 55.8% of cases.

Table II: Distribution of patients according to BOHLER angle

Bohler angle	Number
Positive 25	2
Positive 20	6
Positive 15	9
Positive 10	7
Null	3
Inverted -15	6
Inverted -10	2
Not specified	8
Total	43

14 patients (24.13%) had other associated lesions, mostly lumbar. They were all found in patients with intra-articular fractures.

Table III: Types of associated lesions

Associated lesions	Number
Lumbar	8
Leg	2
Tibial pilon+astragal fracture	1
Tibial pilon fracture	1
Fracture of navicular bone + talus	1
Fracture of the talus	1

I-3: Treatment-Evolution:

All patients underwent open raising and screwing via a lateral approach.

In retrospect, the overall functional outcome was good to excellent in 40 cases (69%). Table V in the analytical section below shows the factors influencing functional outcome.

In concordance with functional results, anatomical results were good to very

good in 16 patients (51%) according to Babin's grading, with a final angle gain
of 16.8° on average.

Complications included delayed healing, superficial sepsis and algodystrophy.
No cases of skin necrosis were reported.

At last recoil, 10% of patients had subtalar osteoarthritis.

Table IV: Differences between thalamic and extra-thalamic fractures

II. Study analytical

	Thalamic Fx (34)	Extra-thalamic Fx (14)	p-value
Age			
[15,35]	20	5	
]36,60]	12	5	0,1
]60,85]	2	4	
Gender			
men	29	10	0,4
women	5	4	
Associated lesions			
yes	11	0	1
no	21	0	
Kitaoka score			
Wrong	3	0	
Medium	19	0	**0,00013**
Good	8	10	
excellent	4	4	

Table V: Factors affecting functional outcome

	Excellent (n=4)	Good (n=6)	Medium (n=21)	Wrong (n=3)	p-value
Age					
[15,35]	2	5	15	3	0,74
]36,60]	2	1	5	0	
]60,85]	0	0	1	0	
Gender					
men	4	6	21	3	1
women	0	0	3	0	
Associated lesions	0	3	10	1	0,4
yes	4	3	14	2	
no					
Duparc					
I	2	3	5	0	0,097
II	0	0	5	0	
III	2	0	2	0	
IV	0	3	6	1	
V	0	0	6	2	
Utheza					
Horizontal	0	0	2	0	**0,015**
Vertical	4	3	4	0	
Mixed	0	3	18	3	

	Excellent (n=4)	Good (n=13)	Medium (n=23)	Wrong (n=3)	p-value
Angle of Bohler	0	0	3	0	
Null	1	3	3	0	
Position at 10	3	3	3	0	
Position at 15	0	4	2	0	
Position at 20	0	0	2	0	0,1
Position at 25	0	1	2	3	
Inversion -15	0	0	2	0	
Inversion -10	0	2	6	0	

DISCUSSION

I. Anatomical and clinical background [2]

The calcaneus is the heel bone. During falls with a hard landing on the heel i0 HVW SUiV HQ WHQDiOOH between the talus and the ground. It undergoes severe shearing contraiQWHV responsible for XQH EDVcXOH GX WKDODPXV (OH WKDODPXV HVW OD SRUWiRQ joint of the top of the calcaneus in contact with the talus).

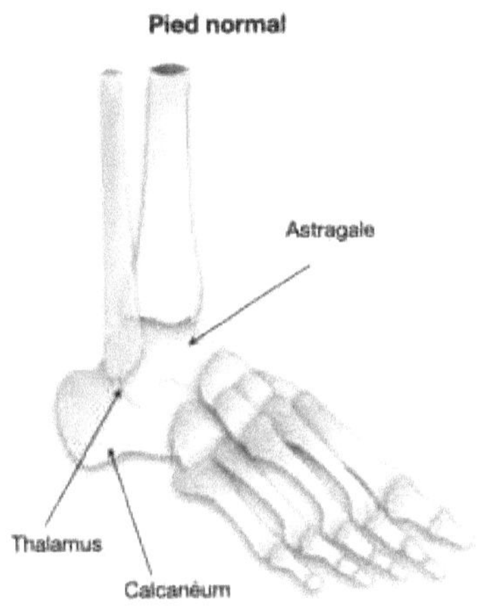

Figure 4: Normal foot

> **Mechanism of injury in calcaneal fractures**

/D IUDcWXUH HVW cDXVéH SDU XQ cKRc YiROHQW VXU OH WDORQ HQWUDiQDQW XQH SUiVH HQ WHQDiOOH of the calcaneus between the ground and the talus

/D IRUWH cRPSUHVViRQ HQJHQGUH XQH EDVcXOH GX WKDODPXV HW XQH IUDJPHQWDWiRQ GX cDOcDQéXP.

*éQéUDOHPHQW, OHV IUDcWXUHV cDOcDQéHQQHV VRQW SURYRTXéHV SDU XQH cKDUJH D[iDOH à KDXWH éQHUJiH VXU OH SiHG (cKXWH GH KDXWHXU VXU OHV WDORQV). (OOHV VRQW VRXYHQW DccRPSDJQéHV

G'DXWUHV EOHVVXUHV JUDYHV ; 10% GHV SDWiHQWV DDQW XQH IUDcWXUH GX cDOcDQéXP SUéVHQWHQW XQH IUDcWXUH WDVVHPHQW WKRUDcR-ORPEDiUH.

/HV IUDcWXUHV GH IDWiJXH SHXYHQW DXVVi VXUYHQiU GDQV OH cDOcDQéXP, SDUWicXOiHUHPHQW cKH] OHV DWKOèWHV HW OHV cRXUHXUV GH ORQJXH GiVWDQcH.

A little anecdote: calcaneal fractures are known as lover's fractures! At the time, the fracture often occurred when a lover jumped from a balcony to avoid detection.

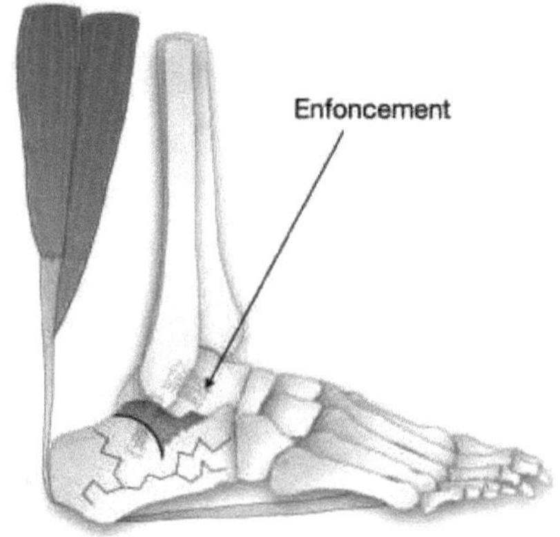

Figure 5: Fractured depression of the calcaneus

Sinking GX WKDODPXV cDOcDQéHQ HQJHQGUH XQH SHUWH cRPSOèWH GH OD cRQJUXHQcH GH the joint with the talus, cHOD cRQGXiUDiW to XQH éURViRQ DUWicXODiUH SURJUHVViYH (DUWKURVH).

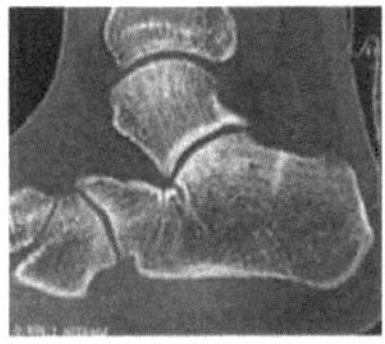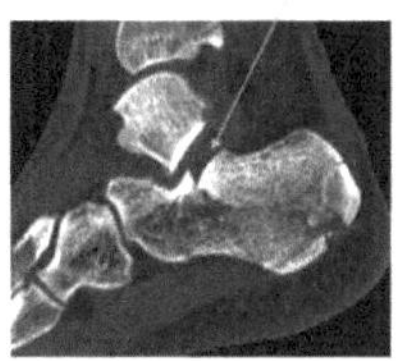

Figure 6: Scans of normal and fractured calcaneus (thalamic depression)

➢ **How is a calcaneal fracture treated?**

- /H WUDiWHPHQW GH IUDcWXUH QRQ-GéSODcéH HVW QRQ cKiUXUJicDO, EDVé VXU XQH PiVH HQ GécKDUJH ViPSOH GH 3 PRiV DYHc XQH UééGXcDWiRQ SUécRcH à OD 3ƒ VHPDiQH.

- 3RXU XQH IUDcWXUH GéSODcéH, OH WUDiWHPHQW HVW cKiUXUJicDO.

- /HV IUDcWXUHV H[WUD DUWicXODiUHV V\PSWRPDWiTXHV VRQW WUDiWéHV SDU 351&((3URWHcWiRQ, 5HVW, IcH, &RPSUHVViRQ, eOéYDWiRQ) followed by an iPPREiOiVDWiRQ SOâWUéH.

- In the absence of a therapeutic consensus, the treatment of DUWicXODiUHV GX cDOcDQéXP UHVWH WRXjRXUV GéOicDW HW VXjHW GH cRQWURYHUVHV fractures. The aim of treatment is to restore anatomy and proper IRQcWiRQQHPHQW GX SiHG. /D PDjRUiWé GHV DXWHXUV RQWcRQcOX à OD VXSéUiRUiWé GX WUDiWHPHQW cKiUXUJicDO SDU UDSSRUW DX WUDiWHPHQW IRQcWiRQQHO, PDiV DYHc XQ UiVTXH DccUX GH cRPSOicDWiRQV. 3OXViHXUV PéWKRGHV WKéUDSHXWiTXHV RQW éWé SURSRVéHV. /H WUDiWHPHQW GH cKRi[SRXU OHV IUDcWXUHV complex remains the reduction and osWéRV\QWKèVH to ciHO RXYHUW, OH WUDiWHPHQW

SHUcXWDQé SHXW êWUH XQH DOWHUQDWiYH YDODEOH SRXU OHV IUDcWXUHV ViPSOHV. /H YiVVDJH GRQQH GHV UéVXOWDWV cRPSDUDEOHV DX WUDiWHPHQW SDU SODTXH.

> ## The rules of surgery

/ intervention begins with OD UéGXcWiRQ GH OD IUDcWXUH SXiV to OD Ii[DWiRQ. IO IDXW éYiGHPPHQW UHVWiWXHU OH SOXV SRVViEOH OHV VXUIDcHV DUWicXODiUHV.

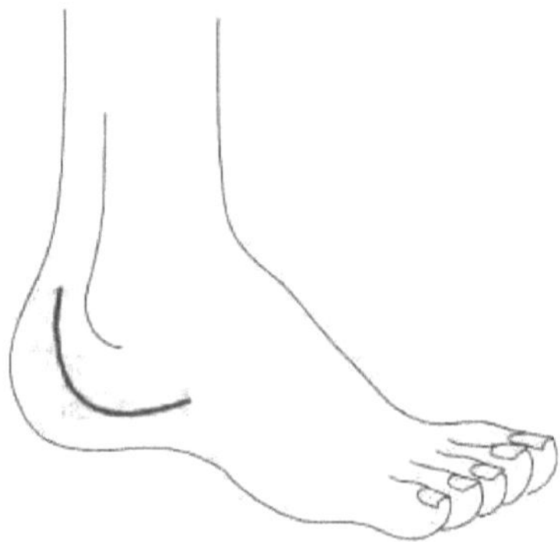

Figure 7: Surgical approach to calcaneal fracture

8QH iQciViRQ DUTXéH à OD SDUWiH H[WHUQH GX SiHG, SHUPHWWDQW to tackle cDOcDQéXP

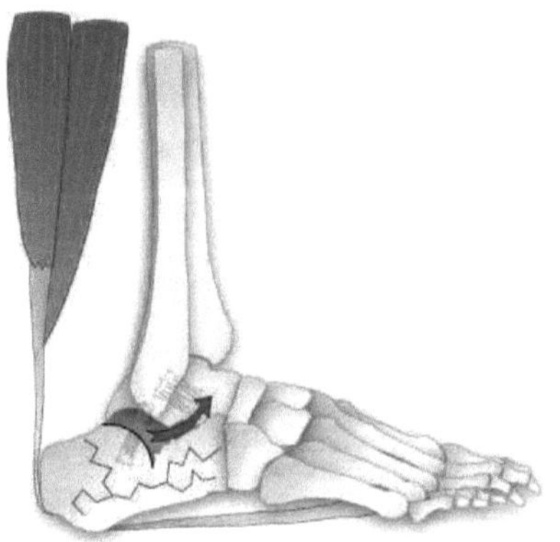

Figure 8: Reconstruction of joint surfaces

$IiQ GH UHcRQVWiWXHU OHV VXUIDcHV DUWicXODiUHV, OH WKDODPXV HVW UHOHYé

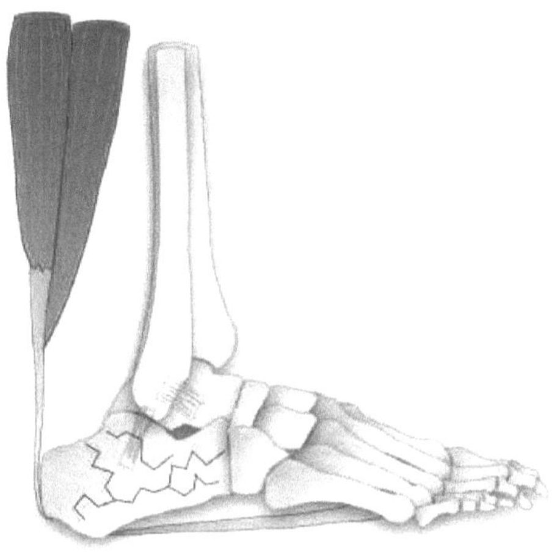

Figure 9: Reduction of calcaneal fracture

The fracture is reduced...

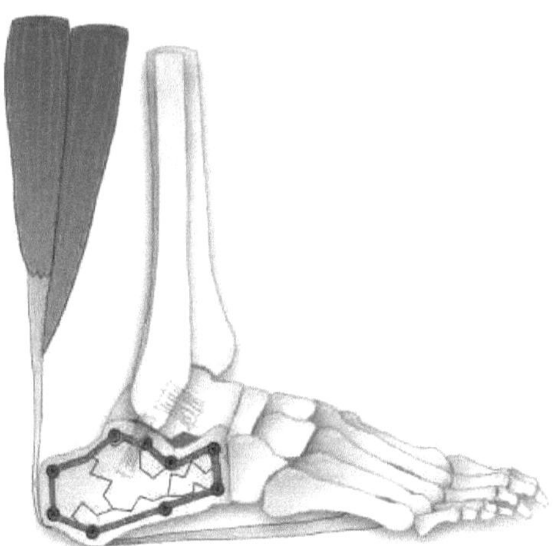

Figure 10: Fixation of calcaneal fracture

CQ IiQ Ii[DWiRQ SDU YiVVHV RX SODTXHV HQ WiWDQH.

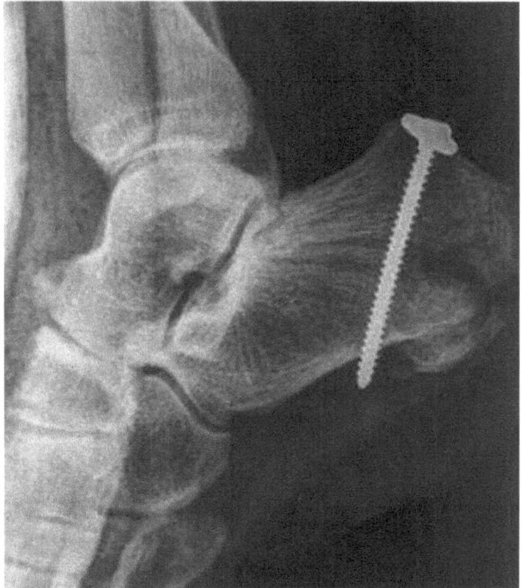

Figure 11: Postoperative radiograph of the calcaneus

II. Our results in relation to literature

Fractures of the calcaneus are among the most dreaded, with extremely long and difficult after-effects. They frequently leave after-effects. A complex calcaneal fracture may take 1 to 2 years to heal properly.

/H WUDiWHPHQW GHV IUDcWXUHV GX cDOcDQéXV D IRUWiRUi WKDODPiTXHV HVW XQ GéIi HW c'HVW VRXYHQW DIIDiUH G'écROH.

Displaced intra-articular calcaneal fractures (DIACF) are the most common type of calcaneal fracture. The differences in therapeutic efficacy between cannulated screw fixation (CSF) and plate fixation are still unclear [7].

The predominance of males has been reported by most authors (men being more exposed) [1,6,8]. Moreover, the age of onset was comparable to that found in the literature [1,6,8]. In fact, this fracture often occurs in young, active subjects, but can also occur in the elderly (in our series, 4 patients had a geriatric age of over 70). In this case, osteoporosis may play a role, and management may be problematic, with a greater impact on autonomy [9].

Thalamic fractures are unique in terms of their mechanism of occurrence, their treatment and their prognosis, which is significantly worse than that of extra-articular fractures. They often require surgical treatment to restore the anatomy of the subtalar joint [1]. In our series, thalamic fractures were predominant (50%) but also mixed in 9% of cases. Approximately 70-75% of fractures are intra-articular, resulting from axial loading, with extra-thalamic fractures being less frequent and less severe [10, 11].

/D OiWWéUDWXUH QRXV iQIRUPH VXU O'iPSRUWDQcH GH O'iQIOXHQcH GHV SDUDPèWUHV GX SDWiHQW (VH[H, âJH, EéQéIicH VHcRQGDiUH) VXU OH UéVXOWDW IRQcWiRQQHO IiQDO [12].

This is often a serious trauma, as evidenced by the frequency of IUDcWXUHV GH W\SH III RX SOXV GH DXSDUc (45%), OH W\SH YHUWicDO IUéTXHQW VHORQ 87+(= (12 YHUWicDO HW 4 KRUi]RQWDO) DiQVi TXH OH QRPEUH GH SDWiHQW SUéVHQWDQW GHV OéViRQV DVVRciéHV (14 SDWiHQWV VRiW 24,13% GRQW 8 cDV DYHc GHV OéViRQV ORPEDiUHV).
/HV VcRUH GH KiWDRND QH GHYUDiW SDV êWUH SHUWXUEé SDV GHV OéViRQV DVVRciéHV QHXURORJiTXHV RX GH O'DSSDUHiO ORcRPRWHXU [9].

Surgery must be preceded by good reduction; in fact, perfectly reduced patients presented a better result than others. Crosby and Fitzgibbons [13] obtained 100% good and very good results for the successful group and 20% for the unsuccessful group. In their view, surgical treatment is essential for all displaced fractures. Currently, most authors report that the treatment of displaced articular fractures of the calcaneus should be surgical [1, 5,7,13].

The operation should be performed as soon as the inflammatory phenomena have resolved by day 7, and the skin incision should be lateralized close to the Achilles tendon. Acute angles should be avoided, dissection should be limited, and the superior flap should be raised from the periosteum, carrying the fibular tendons and sural nerve. The incision should be closed without tension in two planes under drainage [1].

/H WUDiWHPHQW IRQcWiRQQHO HVW cRQViGéUé cRPPH WUDiWHPHQW GH UéIéUHQcH VRXV UéVHUYH G'XQH cRQJUXHQcH JOREDOH GH O'DUWicXODWiRQ VRXV-WDOiHQQH. 8QH RVWéRV\QWKèVH HVW VRXYHQW iQGiTXéH GDQV OHV IUDcWXUHV ViPSOHV à WUDiW IRQGDPHQWDO iQWHUQH DVVRciéHV à XQH YHUWicDOiVDWiRQ GX WKDODPXV ODWéUDO. /'DUWKURGèVH GRiW êWUH UéVHUYéH DX[IUDcDV WKDODPiTXHV [1].

/D WHcKQiTXH GH YiVVDJH H[SRVH à XQ UiVTXH PiQHXU GH cRPSOicDWiRQV cXWDQéHV HW iQIHcWiHXVHV cRQWUDiUHPHQW DX[RVWéRV\QWKèVHV SDU SODTXH R cH UiVTXH SHXW DWWHiQGUH 30% VXUWRXW ORUVTX'iO V'DJiW GH SODTXHV QRQ DGDSWéHV cRPPH cHOD D éWé VRXOiJQé SDU /HYiQ HW 1XQOH\ >14@. /'DGjRQcWiRQ G'XQH JUHIIH RVVHXVH GHPHXUH XQ VXjHW GH GiVcXVViRQ. = iOPRWK >15 @ IXW OH SUHPiHU à SURSRVHU O'DGjRQcWiRQ G'XQH JUHIIH RVVHXVH SRXU cRPEOHU OH YiGH cUé SDU OH UHOèYHPHQW GH OD VXUIDcH WKDODPiTXH. 3DOPHU >16@ D DSSX\é cHWWH iGéH GDQV OH EXW VXSSOéPHQWDiUH GH UHQIRUcHU OD VWDEiOiWé GX UHOèYHPHQW.

DDQV XQH PéWD DQDO\VH cRPSRUWDQW ciQT éWXGHV cRQWU{OéHV UDQGRPiVéHV HW XQ WRWDO GH 707 SDWiHQWV RQW éWé iPSOiTXéV, %DR\RX HW DO >8@ found no GiIIéUHQcH VWDWiVWiTXHPHQW ViJQiIicDWiYH HQWUH OH JURXSH Ii[DWiRQ SDU YiV cDQXOéH HW OH JURXSH Ii[DWiRQ SDU SODTXH HQ WHUPHV G'H[cHOOHQWV HW ERQV VcRUHV $2)$6, DPéiRUDWiRQ GH O'DQJOH GH %RKOHU, DPéiRUDWiRQ GH O'DQJOH GH *iVVDQH, RX OD ODUJHXU GX cDOcDQéXV. 3DU UDSSRUW à OD Ii[DWiRQ SDU SODTXH, iO \ DYDiW XQH UéGXcWiRQ ViJQiIicDWiYH GH OD GXUéH GH OD cKiUXUJiH HW GX WDX[GH cRPSOicDWiRQV. $iQVi, OD Ii[DWiRQ SDU YiVVH cDQXOéH HW OD Ii[DWiRQ SDU SODTXH RQW XQH HIIicDciWé GH Ii[DWiRQ HW GHV UéVXOWDWV IRQcWiRQQHOV ViPiODiUHV GDQV OH WUDiWHPHQW GHV IUDcWXUHV GéSODcéHV iQWUD- DUWicXODiUHV GX cDOcDQéXP. (Q UDiVRQ GH OD GXUéH SOXV cRXUWH GH OD cKiUXUJiH HW GX IDiEOH WDX[GH cRPSOicDWiRQV, OD Ii[DWiRQ SDU YiV cDQXOéH HVW VXSéUiHXUH à OD Ii[DWiRQ SDU SODTXH >8@.

Also in our DDQV study, no relationship was found between associated lesions, Duparc type and Bohler nail on the one hand, and functional outcome on the other; the latter was only statistically significantly correlated with UTH

type(=.

DDQV XQH éWXGH UéWURVSHcWiYH UécHQWH D\DQW cRQcHUQé 98 SDWiHQWV DWWHiQWV GH IUDcWXUHV cDOcDQéHQQHV GH W\SH 6DQGHUV II à III with the aim of éWXGiHU O'HIIHW cOiQiTXH GH OD UéGXcWiRQ SHUcXWDQéH DVVRciéH à OD Ii[DWiRQ iQWHUQH GX cORX cDOcDQéHQ, +XDQJ J HW DO>17@ cRQcOX TXH SDU UDSSRUW à OD UéGXcWiRQ RXYHUWH HW à OD Ii[DWiRQ iQWHUQH, OD UéGXcWiRQ SHUcXWDQéH DVVRciéH à XQ V\VWèPH GH Ii[DWiRQ iQWHUQH GDQV OH WUDiWHPHQW GHV IUDcWXUHV cDOcDQéHQQHV GH W\SH 6DQGHUV II to III HVW UéDOiVDEOH SRXU OD UéSDUDWiRQ GHV IUDcWXUHV VDQV DWWHQGUH OH JRQIOHPHQW GX SiHG, cH TXi SRXUUDiW UHVWDXUHU DYHc SUéciViRQ OD IRUPH HW OD SRViWiRQ QRUPDOHV GH O'RV GX WDORQ IUDcWXUé, éOiPiQHU cRPSOèWHPHQW OH cDO YiciHX[GH OD IUDcWXUH HW UéGXiUH OHV cRPSOicDWiRQV SRVWRSéUDWRiUHV. 3DU cRQVéTXHQW, cHOD SRXUUDiW UDccRXUciU OH WHPSV G'RSéUDWiRQ, OH VéjRXU à O'K{SiWDO, OH WHPSV GH JXéUiVRQ GHV IUDcWXUHV, UéGXiUH OD SHUWH GH VDQJ, IDYRUiVHU OD UécXSéUDWiRQ SRVWRSéUDWRiUH HW PRiQV GH cRPSOicDWiRQV, XQH VécXUiWé éOHYéH, TXi SRXUUDiW êWUH XWiOiVéH cRPPH cKRi[GH cKiUXUJiH RUWKRSéGiTXH SRXU OHV WUDXPDWiVPHV GX SiHG HW GH OD cKHYiOOH >17@.

/D SUiVH HQ cKDUJH GHV IUDcWXUHV cDOcDQéHQQHV iQWUD-DXUicXODiUHV GéSODcéHV (DI$&)) UHVWH GilliciOH HW cRQWURYHUVéH > 18 @. /D UéGXcWiRQ RXYHUWH HW OD Ii[DWiRQ iQWHUQH (25I)) SDU XQH DSSURcKH ODWéUDOH H[WHQViOH RQW éWé ODUJHPHQW DccHSWéHV HW éWDEOiHV cRPPH WUDiWHPHQW VWDQGDUG GHV DI$&) >19,20@. &HSHQGDQW, XQ WDX[DVVH]

éOHYé GH cRPSOicDWiRQV OiéHV à OD SODiH D éWé UDSSRUWé DYHc cHWWH DSSURcKH, QRWDPPHQW XQH QécURVH GX ERUG GH OD SODiH, XQH GéKiVcHQcH, XQ KéPDWRPH, XQH iQIHcWiRQ HW XQH OéViRQ GX QHUI VXUDO >21,22@.

$IiQ GH UéGXiUH OH WDX[GH cRPSOicDWiRQV, GiYHUVHV WHcKQiTXHV PiQi-iQYDViYHV RQW UécHPQW éWé iQWURGXiWHV, QRWDPPHQW OD Ii[DWiRQ H[WHUQH, OD Ii[DWiRQ SHUcXWDQéH, OD Ii[DWiRQ DVViVWéH SDU DUWKURVcRSiH HW OHV WHcKQiTXHV G'iQciViRQ PiQiPDOH SDU YRiH PéGiDOH, ODWéUDOH PRGiIiéH (WHOOH TXH O'DSSURcKH GX ViQXV GX WDUVH), ORQJiWXGiQDOH RX DSSURcKHV cRPEiQéHV >23,24@. &HV WHcKQiTXHV RQW éWé ViJQDOéHV cRPPH HIIicDcHV SRXU PiQiPiVHU OHV WUDXPDWiVPHV GHV WiVVXV PRXV, UéGXiVDQW DiQVi O'iQciGHQcH GHV cRPSOicDWiRQV OiéHV à OD

SODiH.

DDQV OH EXW GH cRPSDUHU OHV UéVXOWDWV IRQcWiRQQHOV HW UDGiRORJiTXHV HW OHV cRPSOicDWiRQV GH OD UéGXcWiRQ SHUcXWDQéH, GH OD Ii[DWiRQ SDU YiV cDQXOéH HW GH OD JUHIIH GH 6&& DYHc cHX[GH O'DSSURcKH PiQi-iQYDViYH GX ViQXV GX WDUVH HW GH OD Ii[DWiRQ SDU SODTXH SRXU OH WUDiWHPHQW GHV DI$&).)HQJ < HW DO >25@ RQW PHQé XQ HVVDi SURVSHcWiI UDQGRPiVé cRQWU{Oé SRUWDQW VXU 80 cDV HW RQW WURXYé TXH OD UéGXcWiRQ SHUcXWDQéH, OD Ii[DWiRQ SDU YiV cDQXOéH HW OD JUHIIH GH &6& SRXU OH WUDiWHPHQW GHV DI$&) 6DQGHUV GH W\SH II SHXYHQW REWHQiU GHV UéVXOWDWV IRQcWiRQQHOV SUHVTXH éTXiYDOHQWV SDU UDSSRUW à O'DSSURcKH PiQiQYDViYH GX ViQXV GX WDUVH HW à OD Ii[DWiRQ SDU SODTXH. /HV GHX[WHcKQiTXHV RQW OHXUV SURSUHV DYDQWDJHV. /D JUHIIH 35+&6& HVW VXSéUiHXUH à OD SURcéGXUH OI67$ HQ WHUPHV GH GéODi PR\HQ HQWUH OD EOHVVXUH iQiWiDOH HW O'RSéUDWiRQ, OD GXUéH GH O'RSéUDWiRQ, OHV cRPSOicDWiRQV OiéHV à OD SODiH HW O'DcWiYiWé GH O'DUWicXODWiRQ VRXV-WDOiHQQH. &HSHQGDQW, OD SURcéGXUH OI67$ D VHV SURSUHV DYDQWDJHV HQ DPéORUDQW OD ODUJHXU cDOcDQéHQQH, HQ IRXUQiVVDQW XQH YiVXDOiVDWiRQ cODiUH HW XQH UéGXcWiRQ SOXV SUéciVH GH OD VXUIDcH DUWicXODiUH, HQ SDUWicXOiHU SRXU OHV DI$&) 6DQGHUV 7\SH-III. /HV UéVXOWDWV IRQcWiRQQHOV GHV DI$&) 6DQGHUV 7\SH-III WUDiWéV SDU OI67$ RQW VXUSDVVé OD JUHIIH 35+&6&.

DDQV QRWUH éWXGH QRXV DYRQV HX UHcRXUV XQiTXHPHQW à OD cRWDWiRQ GH KiWDRND, PDiV QRV UéVXOWDWV IRQcWiRQQHOV éWDiHQW SURcKHV GH cHX[UDSSRUWéV SDU OD OiWWéUDWXUH DYHc

69% GH ERQV à WUèV ERQV UéVXOWDWV. &H UéVXOWDW éWDiW SUiQciSDOHPHQW cRUUéOé DX W\SH
of the thalamic depression, the more vertical the UéVXOWDW HVW ERQ to
H[cHOOHQW.

Anatomical results correlated well with functional results, and were good to very good in 16 patients (51%) according to Babin's grading, with a final angle gain of 16.8° on average.

A meta-analysis of 7 randomized controlled trials involving 902 cases found comparable postoperative functional results between cannulated screw fixation and plate fixation, but there was superiority of cannulated screw fixation over plate fixation in terms of reduction quality, effectiveness time and wound complications >26@.

8QH éWXGH éJ\SWiHQQH SURVSHcWiYH cRPSDUDWiYH HQWUH OHV YiVVHV cDQXOéHV SHUcXWDQéHV HW OHV EURcKHV GH KiUVcKQHU GDQV OH WUDiWHPHQW GHV IUDcWXUHV cDOcDQéHQQHV iQWUD DUWicXODiUHV GéSODcéHV D cRQcOX TXH OHV GHX[WHcKQiTXHV RQW éYiWé OHV cRPSOicDWiRQV GHV SODiHV DVVRciéHV à O'25I), DYHc XQ VéjRXU à O'K{SiWDO SOXV cRXUW. /HV SDWiHQWV GX JURXSH YiVVH cDQXOéH RQW HX GH PHiOOHXUV UéVXOWDWV IRQcWiRQQHOV HW UDGiRORRJiques and an under-WDODiUH SOXV IDiEOH TXH OHV SDWiHQWV GX JURXSH EURcKH GH KiUVcKQHU arthritis rate. /HV YiVVHV cDQXOéHV DYDiHQW OD cDSDciWé GH PDiQWHQiU OD cRUUHcWiRQ REWHQXH HQ SRVWRSéUDWRiUH SOXV TXH OHV EURcKHV GH KiUVcKQHU TXi RQW HQ SOXV O'DYDQWDJH G'XQ WHPSV RSéUDWRiUH UéGXiW SDU UDSSRUW DX[YiVVHV cDQXOéHV HW G'XQH GécKDUJH IDciOH HQ DPEXODWRiUH >27@. /HV DXWHXUV RQW WURXYé TXH /H VHXO IDcWHXU DVVRcié à GH PRiQV ERQV UéVXOWDWV IRQcWiRQQHOV GDQV OHV GHX[JURXSHV éWDiW OH GéYHORSSHPHQW G'XQH DUWKUiWH VRXV-WDOiHQQH.

DDQV QRWUH VéUiH, 10% of patients had subtalar osteoarthritis. Other complications included delayed healing, superficial sepsis and algodystrophy.

A recent Japanese study has once again confirmed the efficacy of HA/PPLA screws (unsintered forged hydroxyapatite and poly-L-lactic acid), with clinical and radiographic results as good as those of plate fixation.

locked in the treatment of intra-articular calcaneal fractures >28@. 3DU DiOOHXUV HQ PDWièUH GH cRPSOicDWiRQV, no skin necrosis or infection was observed in either group. Four patients in group S complained of hindfoot pain, one of whom required arthrodesis of the talocalcaneal joint. One patient in group S required removal of the screw head because of irritating pain. Seven patients in group P require implant removal due to implant irritation and/or hindfoot pain >28@.

DDQV OD OiWWéUDWXUH OH WDX[GHV cRPSOicDWiRQV YDUiH JéQéUDOHPHQW HQWUH 15 HW 25% HW OH WDX[GHV iQIHcWiRQV HQWUH 0.4 HW 27% >29, 30@

III. Limits and self-criticism

- Given the retrospective nature of our study, there was a lack of certain important data, which means that the size of our series is not small compared with other series, but remains relatively acceptable for a mono-centric work. Multicenter randomized controlled trials are needed to derive more scientifically credible and valid results.

-More parameters should have been provided and studied:

- /H cRWé DWWHiQW
- /H PécDQiVPH GH OD IUDcWXUH HW OH OiHX GH WUDXPDWiVPH
- /H WHPSV SDVVé HQWUH WUDXPDWiVPH HW cKiUXUJiH
- /D GXrea of surgery
- /D GXUéH PR\HQQH of hospitalization

-Other scores could have been used to assess functional outcome, e.g. AOFAS (pain, limitation of physical activity, walking surface, gait disorders, sagittal movement, hindfoot movement, etc.).

More rigorous pre- and post-operative parameters for assessing the anatomical result by determining not only the Bohler angle:

- $QJOH GH *iVVDQH
- +DXWHXU GX cDOcDQéXP
- /DUJHXU GX cDOcDQéXP
- /RQJXHXU GX cDOcDQéXP
- 6XUIDcH DUWicXODiUH

CONCLUSION

Calcaneal fractures account for 65% of tarsal fractures, but only 1 to 2% of fractures of the entire skeleton, and are intra-articular in ¾ of cases. It generally occurs in young adults after a fall from a high place, it is painful and leads to significant disability.

While conservative treatment has proved successful for simple fractures, the same cannot be said for complex fractures. Displaced intra-articular calcaneal fractures (DIACF) are the most common type. Open surgical treatment remains the method of choice. Screw fixation is a reliable means of fixation, with good results. The differences in therapeutic efficacy between cannulated screw fixation (CSF) and plate fixation are still unclear.

Today, thanks to a better understanding of anatomical and pathological lesions, and a mastery of the technical bases of open reduction and osteosynthesis of articular fractures of the calcaneus, many authors have reported satisfactory results from surgical treatment.

In our study, conducted with the aim of investigating the functional and anatomical results of facial treatment of calcaneal fractures in the orthopedics-traumatology department at Gafsa regional hospital, we enrolled 58 patients (66 calcaneals), in fact 8 patients had bilateral fractures. The mean age was 38.05 years, with a standard deviation of 16.43 years and extremes ranging from 15 to 85 years. There were 9 women and 49 men, with a sex ratio M/F=5.44. There were 28 extra-thalamic fractures, 34 thalamic fractures and 6 double lesions (thalamic and extra-thalamic). Thalamic depression was vertical in the majority of cases; in fact, the fracture type according to Uthez was horizontal in 4 cases, vertical in 12 cases and mixed in 22 cases, 15 cases being non-typical. The majority of fractures were Duparc type IV and V (35%). The Bohler angle was positive in 55.8% of cases. 14 patients (24.13%)

had other associated lesions, mostly lumbar. They were all noted in patients with intra-articular fractures.

All patients underwent open raising and screw fixation via a lateral approach. We were satisfied with Kitaoka's grading, but overall our functional results were close to those reported in the literature (69% good to very good results). This result was mainly correlated with the type of thalamic depression: the more vertical, the better to excellent the result. Anatomical results correlated with functional results, and were good to very good in 16 patients (51%) according to Babin's grading, with a final gain in angle of 16.8° on average. No relationship was found between associated lesions, Duparc type and Bohler nail on the one hand, and functional result on the other; the latter was only statistically significantly correlated with UTHEZ type. Complications included delayed healing, superficial sepsis and algodystrophy. No cases of skin necrosis were reported. At final follow-up, 10% of patients had subtalar osteoarthritis.

/HV EXWV GX WUDiWHPHQW cKiUXUjicDO GHV IUDcWXUHV DUWicXODiUHV GéSODcéHV GX cDOcDQéXP VRQW WRXjRXUV OH UéWDBEOiVVHPHQW GH O'DQDWRPiH HW OD VXUIDcH DUWicXODiUHH thalamic, obtaining XQ PRQWDJH VWDEOH HW OD OiPiWDWiRQ GHV cRPSOicDWiRQV (cXWDQéH, DUWKURVH VRXV-WDOiHQQH).

CQ UDiVRQ GH OD GXUéH SOXV cRXUWH GH OD cKiUXUJiH HW GX IDiEOH WDX[GH cRPSOicDWiRQV, OD Ii[DWiRQ SDU YiV cDQXOéH HVW VXSéUiHXUH à OD Ii[DWiRQ SDU SODTXH. &HOD SRXUUDiW UDccRXUciU OH WHPSV G'RSéUDWiRQ, OH VéjRXU à O'K{SiWDO, OH WHPSV GH JXéUiVRQ GHV IUDcWXUHV, UéGXiUH OD SHUWH GH VDQJ, IDYRUiVHU OD UécXSéUDWiRQ SRVWRSéUDWRiUH HW PRiQV GH cRPSOicDWiRQV, XQH VécXUiWé éOHYéH, TXi SRXUUDiW êWUH XWiOiVéH cRPPH cKRi[GH cKiUXUJiH RUWKRSéGiTXH SRXU OHV WUDXPDWiVPHV GX SiHG HWGH OD cKHYiOOH.

Further studies are needed to evaluate cannulated screw fixation for different types of Sanders calcaneal fractures.

REFERENCES

1. (O$ODPi %, 1DDP, $GPi 0, 5DEKi I, (OEDUGDi 0, %RXWD\HE). 7UDiWHPHQW cKiUXUicD0 GHV IUDcWXUHV GX cDOcDQéXP : à SURSRV GH 29 cDV. Pan Afr Med J. 2017; 26: 137.

2. /DSiHUUH %.)UDcWXUH GX cDOcDQéXP. KWWSV://U.VHDUcK.\DKRR.cRP/ ZZZ.GUERYiHU-ODSiHUUH.IU.IUDcWXUH-GX-cDOcDQHXP.

3. DXSDUc J, &DIIiQièUH J<. 0écDQiVPH, DQDWRPRSDWKRORJiH, cODVViIicDWiRQ GHV IUDcWXUHV DUWicXODiUHV GX cDOcDQéXP. *Ann Chir.* 1970 0DU; 24(5):289-301.

4. KiWDRND +%, $OH[DQGHU IJ, $GHODDU 56, 1XQOH\ J$, 0\HUVRQ 06, 6DQGHUV O. &OiQicD0 UDWiQJ V\VWHPV IRU WKH DQNOH-KiQGIRRW, PiGIRRW, KDOOX[, DQG OHVVHU WRHV. *Foot Ankle Int.* 1994 JX0; 15(7):349-53.

5. %DEiQ 65, *UDI 3, KDW]QHU O, 6cKYiQJW (. 6cUHZHG-SODWH RVWHRV\QWKH ViV DQG UHcRQVWUXcWiRQ RI IUDcWXUHV RI WKH cDOcDQHXV. *Rev Chir Orthop Reparatrice Appar Mot.* 1982; 68(8):557-69.

6. /XR *,)DQ &, *DR 3, +XDQJ =, 1i =. $Q HYDOXDWiRQ RI WKH HIIicDc\ RI SHUcXWDQHRXV UHGXcWiRQ DQG VcUHZ Ii[DWiRQ ZiWKRXW ERQH JUDIWiQJ iQ 6DQGHUV Type-II and Type-III displaced intra-articular calcaneal fractures. %0& 0XVcXORVNHOHWDO DiVRUGHUV (2022) 23:562.

7. %DR\RX (, =KRX ;, =Hi =, <iPiQJ 5, /iQ =, +DR < HW DO.)i[DWiRQ SDU YiV cDQDXOéH HW Ii[DWiRQ SDU SODTXH SRXU IUDcWXUH GX cDOcDQéXP iQWUD-DUWicXODiUH GéSODcéH : XQH PéWD-DQDO\VH G'HVVDiV cRQWU{OéV UDQGRPiVéV. IQW. J 6XUJ 2016 Oct; 34:64-72.

8. 6D\HG-+RVVHiQiDQ 6, 6KiDUD]iDQ 0, $UDEi +, $IIDO $JKDHH 0, :DKHGi (, %DJKHUi). DRHV WKH SRVWRSHUDWiYH TXDOiW\ RI UHGXcWiRQ, UHJDUGOHVV RI WKH VXUJicD0 method used in treating a calcaneal fracture, influence patients' functional RXWcRPHV " %0& 0XVcXORVNHOHWDO DiVRUGHUV (2023) 24:562

9. Kuntz JK, Sibilia J, Durckel J, Kieffer D, Meyer R, Asch L. Spontaneous calcaneal fracture in the elderly without fluoride treatment. Rev Rhum Mal

Ostéoartique 1989 novembre ; 56(11) :759-61.

10. 3HQJ <, ꞊DQJ J,)HQJ %, /i <, =KX <, <XDQ ꞊ HW DO. &DOcDQHRXV iQWHUORRcNiQJ QDiO WUHDWPHQW IRU cDOcDQHRXV IUDcWXUH: D PXOWiSOH cHQWHU UHWURVSHcWiYH VWXG\. 3HQJ et al. BMC Musculoskeletal Disorders (2022) 23:911

11. DDIWDU\ $, +DiPV $.+, %DXPJDHUWQHU 0.5,)UDcWXUHV RI WKH cDOcDQHXV: D UHYiHZ ZiWK HPSKDViV RQ &7, 5DGiRJUDSKicV 25 (2005) 1215-1226.

12. Roussignol X, Cavalhana G, Polle G, Duparc F, Dujardin F. eYDOXDWiRQ GHV UéVXOWDWV GX WUDiWHPHQW IRQcWiRQQHO HWcKiUXUJicDO GHV IUDcWXUHV WKDODPiTXHV GX cDOcDQéXV : à SURSRV G'XQH VéUiH UéWURVSHcWiYH GH 304 cDV. 0éGHciQH HW &KiUXUJiH GX 3iHG 2012 (28) :15-23.

13. Crosby LA, Fitzgibbons TC. Open reduction and osteosynthesis of type II intra-articular calcaneal fractures. Foot Ankle Int.1996 May ;17 (5):253-8.

14. Levin LS, Nunley JA. The management of soft tissue problems associated with calcaneal fractures. Clin Orthop Relat Res. 1993 May;(290):151-6.

15. Wilmoth P. Treatment of calcaneal fractures. J de Med et Chir Prat. 1931 ; 102: 328-35.

16. Palmer I. The mechanism and treatment of calcaneal fractures. J Bone Joint Surg Am. January 1948; 30A (1) :2-8.

17. Huang J, Liu J, Zhang J. Treatment of Sanders-type calcaneal fractures II to III with percutaneous reduction and minimally invasive calcaneal screw fixation. Zhongguo Gu Shang.2023; 36(4):313-9.

18. 5DPPHOW 6, =ZiSS +. &DOcDQHXV IUDcWXUHV: IDcWV, cRQWURYHUViHV DQG UHcHQW GHYHORSPHQWV. IQjXU\. 2004; 35:443-61.

19. 6DQGHUV 5. DiVSODcHG iQWUD-DUWicXODU IUDcWXUHV RI WKH cDOcDQHXV. J %RQH JRiQW 6XUJ $P. 2000; 82:225-50.

20. %XcNOH\ 5, 7RXJK 6, 0c&RUPDcN 5, 3DWH *, /HiJKWRQ 5, 3HWUiH D, HW DO. 2SHUDWiYH cRPSDUHG ZiWK QRQRSHUDWiYH WUHDWPHQW RI GiVSODcHG iQWUDDUWicXODU iQWUDDUWicXODU cDOcDQHDO IUDcWXUHV: D SURVSHcWiYH, UDQGRPi]HG, cRQWUROOHG

PXOWicHQWHU WUiDO. J %RQH ßiQW 6XUJ $P. 2002; 84:1733-44.

21. +RZDUG J/, %XcNOH\ 5, 0c&RUPDcN 5, 3DWH *, /HiJKWRQ 5, 3HWUiH D, HW DO. &RPSOicDWiRQV **IROORRZiQJ** PDQDJHPHQW RI GiVSODcHG iQWUD-DUWicXODU cDOcDQHDO IUDcWXUHV : D SURVSHcWiYH UDQGRPi]HG WUiDO cRPSDUiQJ RSHQ UHGXcWiRQ iQWHUQDO Ii[DWiRQ ZiWK QRQRSHUDWiYH PDQDJHPHQW. J 2UWKRS 7UDXPD. 2003; 17:241-9.

22. $0-0XGKDIIDU **O**, 3UDVDG &9, 0RIiGi $. ᴢRXQG cRPSOicDWiRQV IROORRZiQJ RSHUDWiYH Ii[DWiRQ RI cDOcDQHDO IUDcWXUHV. IQjXU\. 2000; 31:461-4.

23. 5DPRV 55, GH &DVWUR)iOKR &D, 5DPRV 55, %iWWDU &K, GH &iOOR 06, GH ODWWRV &$, HW DO. 6XUJicDO WUHDWPHQW RI iQWUD-DUWicXODU cDOcDQHDO IUDcWXUHV: GHVcUiSWiRQ RI D WHcKQiTXH **XV/iQJ** DQ DGjXVWDEOH XQiSODQDU H[WHUQDO Ii[DWRU. 6WUDWHJiHV 7UDXPD /iPE 5HcRQVWU. 2014; 9:163-6.

24. =KDQJ 7, 6X <, &KHQ ᴢ, =KDQJ 4, ᴢX =, =KDQJ <. DiVSODcHG iQWUDDUWicXODU cDOcDQHDO IUDcWXUHV WUHDWHG iQ D PiQiPDOO\ iQYDViYH IDVKiRQ:ORQJiWWXGiQDO DSSURDcK YHUVXV ViQXV WDUVi DSSURDcK. J %RQH JRiQW 6XUJ $P. 2014 ; 96:302-9.

25.)HQJ <, 6KXi ;, ᴢDQJ J, &Di /, <X <, <iQJ ᴢ HW DO. &RPSDUDiVRQ GH OD Ii[DWiRQ SDU YiV cDQXOéH SHUcXWDQéH HW GH OD JUHIIH GH ciPHQW DX VXOIDWH GH cDOciXP SDU UDSSRUW à O'DSSURcKH PiQi-iQYDViYH GX ViQXV GX WDUVH HW à OD Ii[DWiRQ SDU SODTXH SRXU OHV IUDcWXUHV cDOcDQéHQQHV iQWUD-DUWicXODiUHV GéSODcéHV : XQ HVVDi SURVSHcWiI UDQGRPiVé cRQWWU{Oé. <u>7URXEOH PXVcXORVTXHOHWWiTXH %O&.</u> 2016; 17: 288.

26. ᴢDQJ 4, =KDQJ 1, *XR ᴢ, ᴢDQJ ᴢ, =KDQJ 4. &DQQXODWHG VcUHZ Ii[DWiRQ versus plate fixation in treating displaced intra-articular calcaneus fractures: a systematic review and meta-analysis. International Orthopaedics (2021) 45:2411- 2421.

27. (O-$]DE +, $KPHG K, KKDOHID $, **ODUU**]RXN $. $ SURVSHcWiYH cRPSDUDWiYH VWWXG\ EHWZHHQ SHUcXWDQHRXV cDQQXODWHG VcUHZV DQG KiUVcKQHU ZiUHV iQ WUHDWPHQW of displaced intra-articular calcaneal fractures. International Orthopaedics (2022) 46:2667-2683.

28. 8VDPi 7, 7DNDGD 1, liVKiGD K, 6DNDi +, IZDWD +, <RQHVX + HW DO.)i[DWiRQ RI iQWUD-DUWicXODU cDOcDQHDO IUDcWXUHV : $ cRPSDUDWiYH VWXG\ RI WKH SRVWRSHUDWiYH RXWcRPH EHWZHHQ +$/33/$ VcUHZV DQG ORcNiQJ SODWHV. +HOi\RQ 9 (2023) H14046.

29. 6cKXEHUWK JO, &REE 0D, 7DODUicR 5+. 0iQiPDOO\ iQYDViYH DUWKURVcRSic- DVViVWHG UHGXcWiRQ ZiWK SHUcXWDQHRXV Ii[DWiRQ iQ WKH PDQDJHPHQW RI iQWUD-DUWicXODU cDOcDQHDO IUDcWXUHV: D UHYiHZ RI 24 cDVHV. J)RRW $QNOH 6XUJ. 2009; 48:315-22.

30. %iJJi), Di)DEiR 6, D'$QWiPR &, IVRQi), 6DOIi &, 7UHYiVDQi 6. 3HUcXWDQHRXV cDOcDQHRSODVW\ iQ GiVSODcHG iQWUDDUWicXODU cDOcDQHDO IUDcWXUHV. J 2UWKRS 7UDXPDWRO. 2013 ; 14:307-10.

APPENDICES

Appendix 1: Measuring the Bohler angle

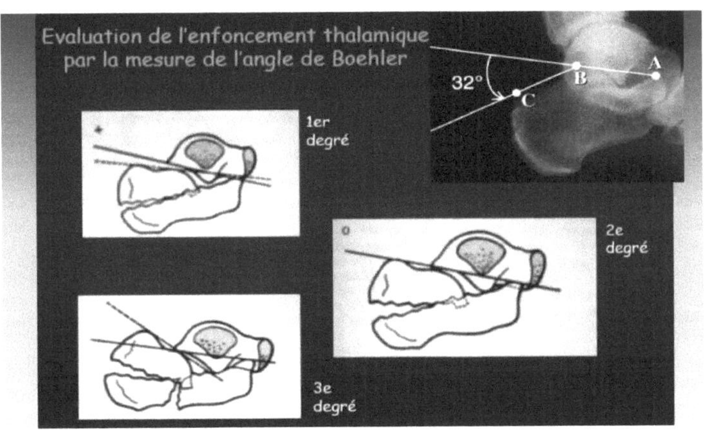

Appendix 2: UTHEZA classification

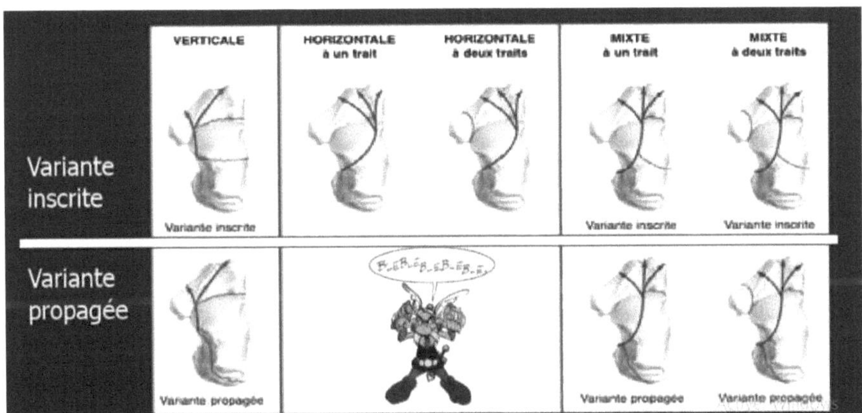

Appendix 3: SANDERS classification

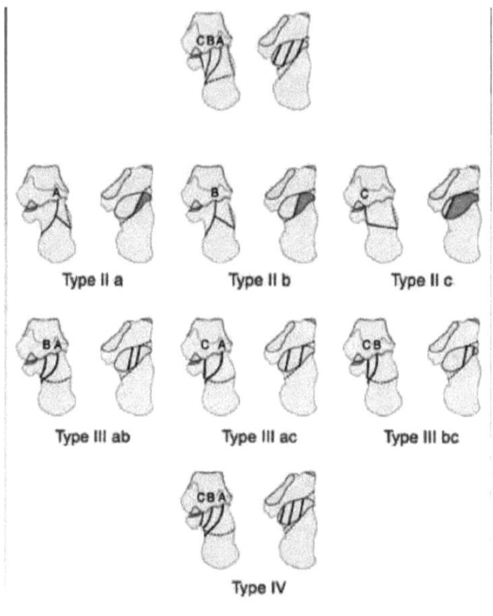

Monastir Faculty of Medicine

Academic year 23/24

Dissertation for the CEC PODOLOGIE N° ...

Title: Evaluation of screw treatment of calcaneal fractures in Gafsa

---

Summary

Calcaneal fractures account for 65% of tarsal fractures, but only 1 to 2% of fractures of the entire skeleton, and are intra-articular in ¾ of cases. It often occurs in young adults after a fall from a high place, is painful and leads bsignificant disability. Displaced intra-articular calcaneal fractures (DIACF) are the most common type. Open surgical treatment remains the method of choice. Screw fixation is a reliable means of fixation, with good results. The differences in therapeutic efficacy between cannulated screw fixation (CSF) and plate fixation are not yet known.

unclear.

Our aim was to study the functional and anatomical results of facial treatment of calcaneal fractures in the orthopedics department at Gafsa regional hospital. We collected 58 patients (66 calcaneals), 8 patients had bilateral fractures. Theaverage age was 38 years (15-85 years). There were 9 women and 49 men (sex ratio M/F=5.44). There were 28 extra-thalamic fractures, 34 thalamic and 6 double lesions (thalamic and extra-thalamic). Thalamic depression was vertical in the majority of cases, and the type of fracture according to Uthez was horizontal in 4 cases, vertical in 12 cases and mixed in 22 cases, 15 cases being untyped. The majority of fractures were Duparc type IV and V (35%). The Bohler angle was positive in 55.8% of cases. 14 patients (24.13%) had other associated lesions, mostly lumbar. They were all noted in patients with intra-articular fractures.

All patients underwent open raising and screw fixation via a lateral approach. According to the Kitaoka grading system, our functional results were comparable to those reported in the literature, with 69% good to very good results. This result was mainly correlated with the type of thalamic recess, the more vertical the recess, the better to excellent the result. Anatomical results correlated with functional results, and were good to very good in 16 patients (51%) according to Babin's grading, with a final gain in angle of 16.8° on average. No relationship was found between associated lesions, Duparc type and Bohler nail on the one hand, and functional result on the other; the latter was significantly correlated only with UTHEZ type. Complications included delayed healing, superficial sepsis and algodystrophy. There were no cases of skin necrosis, and 10% of patients had subtalar osteoarthritis.

Key words: Fracture, calcaneus, thalamic, Bohler, Duparc, Screwing,

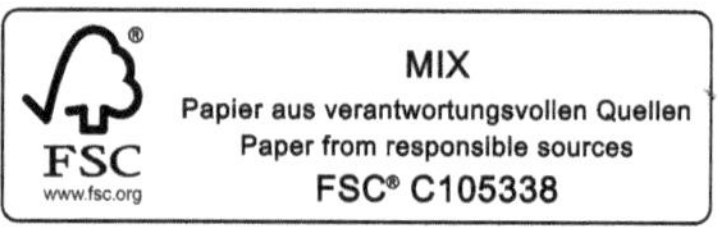

Printed by Books on Demand GmbH, Norderstedt / Germany